Mouth Wide Open

How To Ask Intelligent Questions About Dental Implants and Make Empowered Choices from the Answers

Steven J. Brazis, DDS

ISBN: 0692728406

Table of Contents

Acknowledgements

I wish to acknowledge my family for putting up with me during the writing of this book. The many times they wanted to spend time with me and had to hear: "I have to get this done—I have a deadline." It is done and I am back. Thank you so much for your faith and patience. I also would like to acknowledge my good friend, David McKay. David is a master photographer and author himself. David led me to the Self-Publishing School after experiencing success with his release of "Photography Demystified: Your Guide to Gaining Creative Control and Taking Amazing Photographs." The Self-Publishing School has been an enormous help and resource during the process of getting this book to you.

I also would like to acknowledge my professional friends who have helped by supplying their insight and knowledge. Mark Zablotsky, DDS, my long term friend, photography buddy, and respected periodontist, who wrote the editorial review for Amazon. Mark has treated many of my patients in the surgical aspect of implant placements as well as treating their periodontal disease, and does a lot of educating himself, both personally and through his study club. Sean Rhee, another periodontist and good friend, who has treated my patients surgically and spent much time consulting with me on case planning. Shama Currimbhoy, DDS, an oral surgeon who invited me to participate in a series of lectures on implant dentistry given by her office for dentists in Sacramento and who has also been a friend and consultant on many cases. There are too many to list here, but I thank all my professional friends not only for any direct input they may have had over the years, but also for their own dedication to their profession and to their patients. They raise the bar for me constantly.

I also need to acknowledge all of the patients who have stuck with me over the years, trusting me with their dental treatment and the dental well-being of their families. I am blessed with a rich cross section of patients from many walks of life and I am honored by their trust and their loyalty. Without them there would be no book and, indeed, I would have no dental practice. You are all the best and my appreciation is boundless.

Introduction

I will tell you the answers to the questions mentioned in the table of contents in this book. Some of the questions will be answered together as they are closely related. Each question, or combination of questions, will comprise a chapter of this book. The chapters can be read in order or you can go directly to the section containing the answers you are most interested in. The answers will make sense and be easy to understand, but they are not a treatment plan. The purpose of this book is to provide the kind of information that will enable you to have an intelligent conversation with your own dentist about your treatment plan, empowering you to be proactive in making the decisions about your own dental treatment plan with respect to implants.

There is also a bonus question that I am going to pose here. It is the most important question of all, but so often overlooked. It is not a question I can answer, nor can your dentist. The question: "Do I Want Dental Implants?" All the above questions are really about knowing what implants are, whether they work, and whether they would work for you.

These are the kinds of questions that we as dentists excel at answering, and we tend to assume that when you get satisfactory answers to the questions, you will feel the same way we do. If anyone were to ask me if I think implants work or are they a good alternative or do I like to do implants, my answer is: I love implants. I could do dental implants all day long. But I'm not the one who has to go through the treatment or live with them.

I can't answer this question for you, but I will address the question again at the end of the book and hopefully give you some food for thought about your own point of view that perhaps you haven't considered or heard before.

I am a general/restorative dentist. I graduated from the University of the Pacific School of Dentistry in 1973. I opened my first practice in San Francisco in the well-known 450 Sutter medical/dental building in downtown San Francisco, across from Union Square. In those early days of my career, we were still using silver amalgam as the main filling material; bonding was something you did with a family member and implants were a research concept. The personal computer revolution was still a future development, and the concept of the Internet was just being developed by the military but unheard of in the general public.

To be a dentist during these years has been my great privilege and joy. The fields of medicine and dentistry have seen more advancement in technology and materials science during the last 40-50 years than at any other time in history. I will spend a few minutes on this here because these developments in computer technology were essential to the development and state of the art currently in dental implants.

In the late 1970's, I was introduced to my first computer by a good friend, Carlos Berguido, who was himself an electronics genius. The computer was a tiny little box put out by Timex Corporation. It had to be plugged into a TV set for a monitor. It could accept DOS commands (Disc Operating System) and I had my first exposure to writing basic DOS programs. Today, very few people even remember or ever heard of DOS.

Later, in the late 1980's, personal computers started to become more common and, deciding I did not want to be left behind the curve of technological progress, I went out and bought an IBM 8086 computer. It came with two 5½-inch floppy disc drives, a monitor and a keyboard. No hard drive. I later added my first hard drive—20 whopping kilobytes. Thought I would never fill that up. TBT, LOL, LMAO and other modern acronyms weren't around then, but LMAO!!

After that it was a blitz. The 8086 became the 80286, the 80386, and then Windows came along. That's when multitasking became possible and computers began to really take over the world. I was very glad for my early programming escapades because that gave me an edge to handle the increasingly computerized developments in technology everywhere, including dentistry.

Then the onset of digital imaging really made a huge difference. That's when CAT scans and CBCT scans became possible, initiating development of technology-driven solutions in medicine and dentistry that made the current state of dental implant therapy possible. The CAT scan (computed axial tomography scan) is a means of taking a series of digital images of body tissues and using a computer algorithm to put them together to render an image that gives the 3-dimensional relationships of tissues (bone, nerves, soft tissue) in the area scanned. CBCT stands for cone beam computed tomography. This is a specialized version of a CAT scan that has become so useful in dental application, particularly in the field of dental implants.

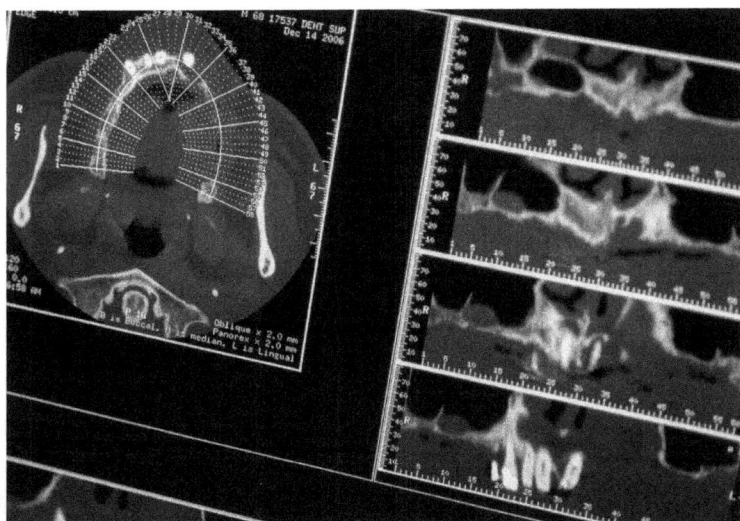

At the same time all this was taking place, the concept of bonded restorations, using composite resin materials, was rapidly advancing. Bond strengths were improving, esthetic qualities of the composites and ceramic porcelains were improving, and the scope of bonding was widening to include the cements we use (among many other uses).

In my current practice in Sacramento, CA, I am the grateful recipient of many years of dedicated research and development in dental technology, and my patients are the final recipients of all this development. It is my pleasure to write this book to give you, the reader, an idea how all this technology can bring you the benefit of superior tooth replacement options in the form of dental implants and dental implant supported restorations.

What Are Dental Implants and What Are They Made Of?

These two questions are closely related and are usually the first questions that patients ask me when faced with a possible treatment of dental implants. In this chapter, I will discuss what implants are, how they are structured, and what materials are used in the various parts of an implant case. Knowing these things and being able to visualize the parts is the first step in being able to see how implants can serve you.

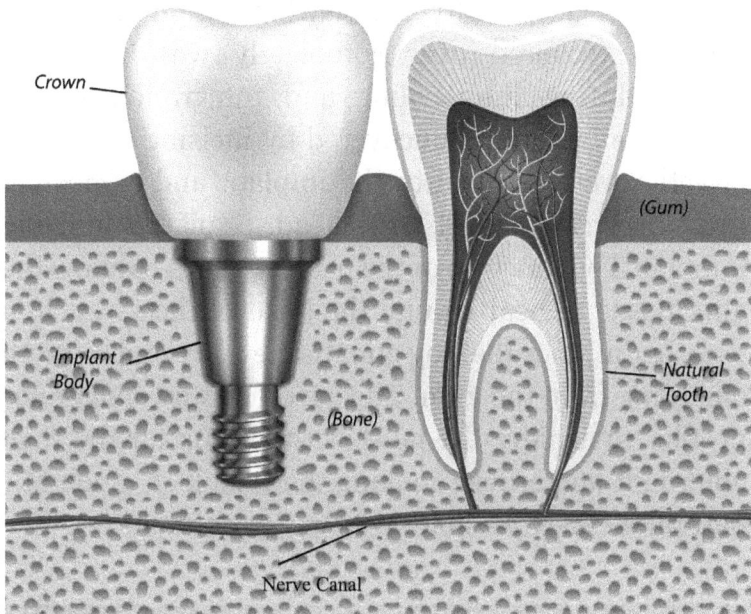

Crown — Implant Body — (Gum) — Natural Tooth — (Bone) — Nerve Canal

What Are Implants

An implant is an artificial tooth root surgically placed in the jawbone to substitute for a missing tooth. Usually patients think of an implant as the whole tooth, filling in the space where the missing tooth was. Technically, though, the implant is the root portion of the tooth surgically placed in the bone. After being placed, a variable amount of healing time is allowed for the implant to become integrated with the bone of the jaw so that it is stable enough to support the biting and chewing stresses after restoration is completed.

During the surgical phase of treatment, the implant body is placed into the jawbone and generally "buried" (covered over completely with the gum tissue) during the healing and integration phase. Later, the implant is uncovered by incising the tissue directly over the head of the implant and a "healing cap," or screw with a large head, is placed into the implant. The function of the healing cap is to allow the gum tissue to heal around the head of the screw in a way that mimics the way gum tissue surrounds a tooth emerging from the gum. This gives us our "emergence profile" to achieve the most natural look for the final abutment and crown, making them look as much like natural teeth as possible.

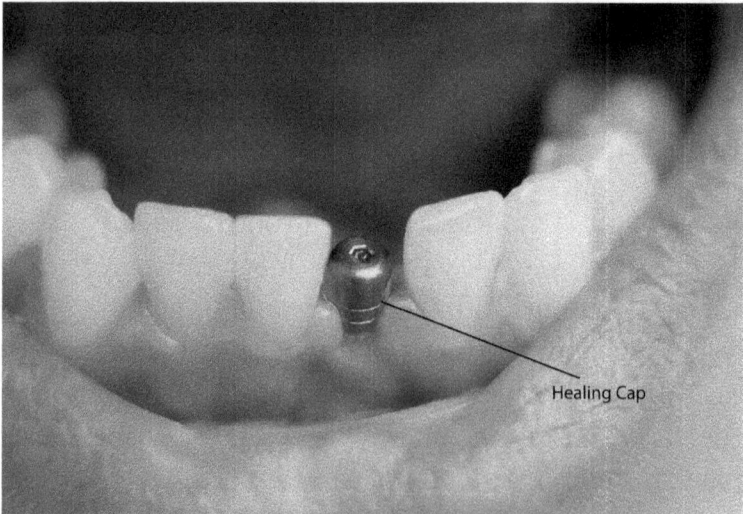

Healing Cap

(This picture shows a healing cap for a lower front tooth—a stayplate can be made to cover this with a plastic tooth)

How Are Implants Structured

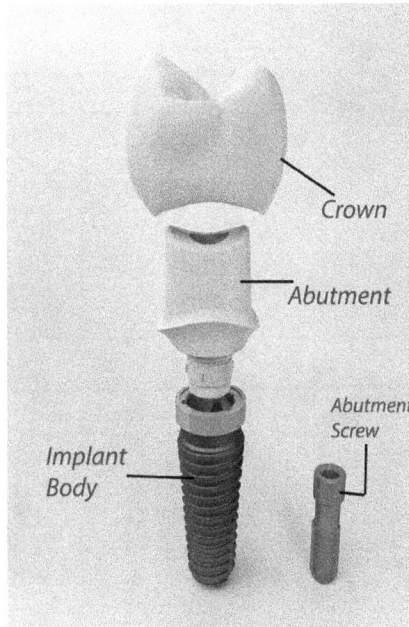

Crown

Abutment

Abutment Screw

Implant Body

The completion of the process involves screwing a piece called an abutment into the implant, then cementing a crown over the abutment. These are done at the same time and take the same amount of time to complete as a regular crown on a tooth.

If multiple implants are being done, the process is the same but may take longer if the implant sites are in different areas in the mouth. If multiple teeth are missing in the same area, each tooth does not necessarily require a corresponding implant. Implants can be placed at both ends of a longer "gap" and a fixed bridge placed on them, just like on teeth with a gap between them.

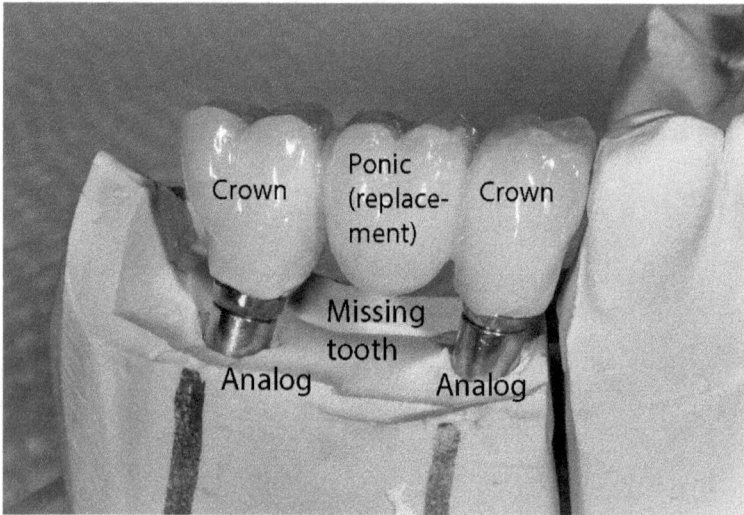

If a removable denture is used to replace multiple missing teeth, the implants that are placed to stabilize the denture will get a different type of abutment screwed into them, called attachments. There are many types of these attachments available, and they will mate with a receptor part which is built into the denture base. When the denture is seated in the mouth, it will "snap" into place on the attachments and become very stable.

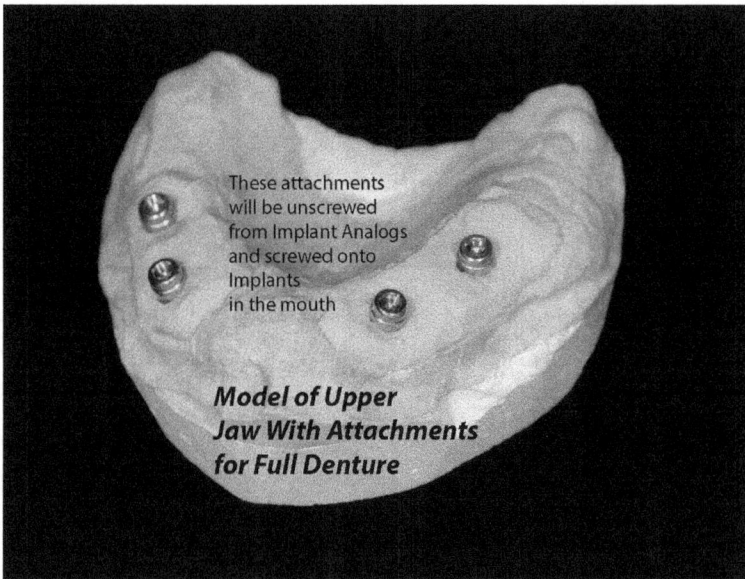

These attachments will be unscrewed from Implant Analogs and screwed onto Implants in the mouth

Model of Upper Jaw With Attachments for Full Denture

What Materials Are Used

Implants are most commonly made from titanium or a titanium alloy. Titanium is a biocompatible metal, meaning it is not rejected by the body. Implants can also be coated with a form of hydroxyapatite, a naturally occurring ingredient in bone and tooth structure that is said to enhance osseointegration, the ability of bone to fuse to the implant surface. Osseointegration is the basis for dental implant success and is the reason for the long delay between surgical placement of the implant and the placement of the abutment and final tooth (or teeth) restoration on top of the implant(s). The dental surgeon who places the implant will monitor the site at intervals and test the implant for stability to determine when to pronounce the implant "ready for restoration."

The abutment portion of the implant process can be made of titanium, a dental gold alloy, or zirconium (a ceramic material). The abutments can be preformed or custom made by the dental laboratory. Custom abutments are used to re-align the abutment to the long axis of the adjacent teeth when the implant body is significantly out of alignment with the teeth. This happens because the jaw ridge the implant is placed in is at an angle to the teeth emerging from it. This is most common in the upper front area where the upper jaw tends to angle forward to provide support for the lip, but the front teeth angle downward to provide incision action with the lower front teeth.

There are many factors involved in choosing an implant placement site and angulation, which makes the use of custom abutments a very common necessity. Implant placement sites are affected not only by the angle of jawbone, but also by the angle of the natural tooth roots of adjacent teeth, presence of the sinus cavity, nerve canals and foramen nearby, and thickness of the jawbone, among others. These factors are all part of the implant treatment planning process and should be jointly considered by the surgeon and the restorative dentist. Implants can be a team effort by a separate surgeon and restorative (often called "general") dentist, or they can be done by a restorative dentist with surgical training as well as specialized implant placement surgical training (someone who can perform the whole process alone).

The crown or fixed bridge placed on top of the abutments are made from the same materials that crowns placed on natural teeth are made from. Gold, porcelain fused to a gold-platinum-palladium alloy, and porcelain (ceramic) are the usual choices. The choice of material to use is usually a matter of considering strength versus esthetics. Although ceramic alternatives are a given in replacement of front teeth, today's ceramic materials are so much improved over the ceramics of previous decades that the use of ceramic materials to make back teeth more esthetic is quite common.

Finally, the attachments used to stabilize removable denture appliances are generally a preformed, titanium alloy (of various sizes and types), and will usually be decided upon by collaboration between the restorative dentist and the laboratory technician who makes the denture.

Once the implant body has fully integrated with the bone and become stable enough to "restore" (have the abutment and crown placed), the dentist doing the restorative portion will need two parts in order to continue. He will need an analog implant and an impression coping. The analog implant will be incorporated into the stone model on which the final abutment and crown are made by the dental laboratory. This analog represents the implant body which is now in your jawbone.

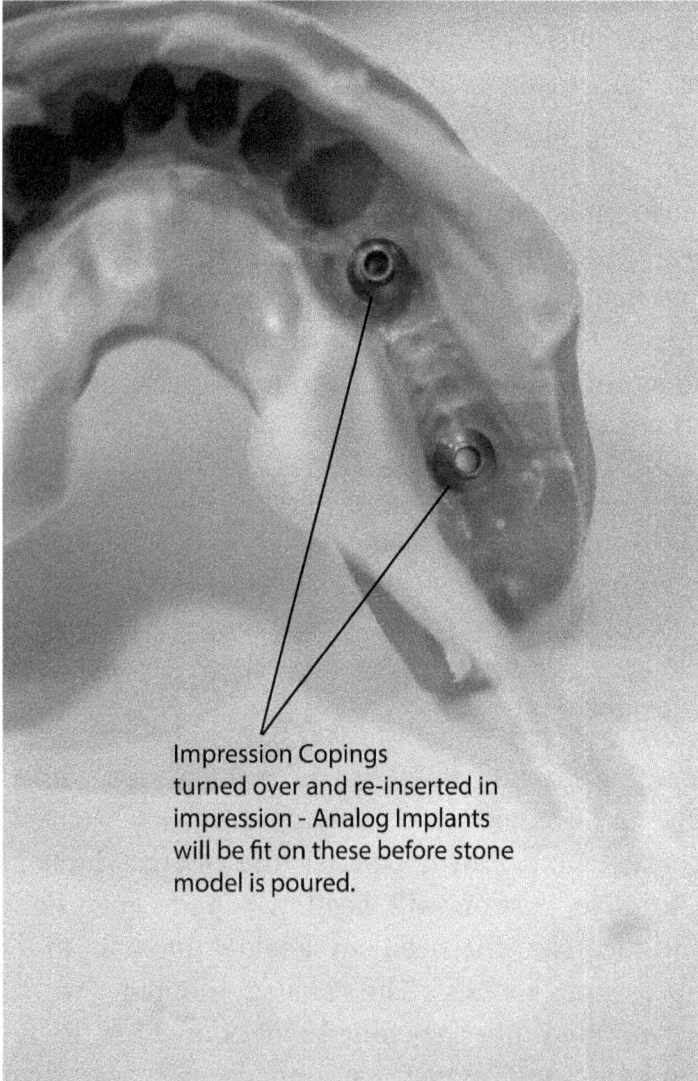

Impression Copings turned over and re-inserted in impression - Analog Implants will be fit on these before stone model is poured.

In order to ensure that the exact position and angulation of the analog implant in the model matches that of the implant body in your jaw, an impression coping is screwed into the implant body in your jaw. This usually requires unscrewing the piece placed by the surgeon (the healing cap). It is nothing more than a screw with a large "head" that protrudes from the implant body, which is below the level of the soft tissue (gums), into the mouth high enough to be surrounded by impression material when an impression of the jaw, all the remaining teeth and soft tissue, as well as the coping, is taken.

After the impression is removed from the mouth, the impression coping can be unscrewed, turned over, and re-inserted into the impression. The dental laboratory then takes the analog implant and screws it onto the impression coping sticking up from the impression. The whole thing then has dental stone poured into it, creating a model of your teeth containing an analog implant in the same position and angle as the implant body already in your jaw.

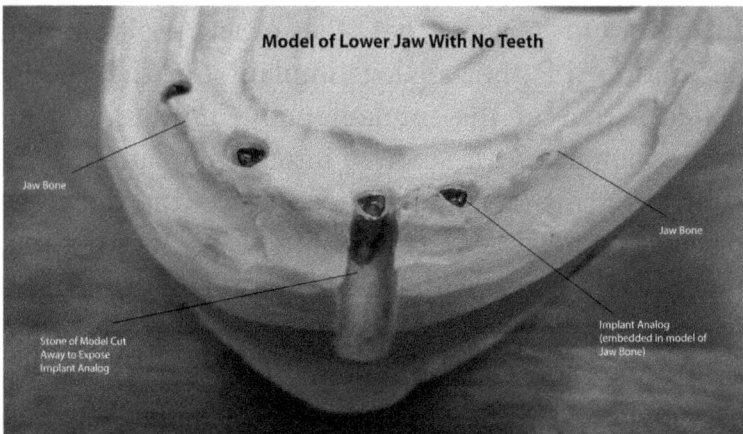

Model of Lower Jaw With No Teeth

Jaw Bone

Jaw Bone

Stone of Model Cut Away to Expose Implant Analog

Implant Analog (embedded in model of Jaw Bone)

Now the laboratory can fit an abutment and build a crown (or bridge or fit an attachment for a denture). The healing cap screw is replaced after the impression is removed and a separate "bite" impression taken to allow the laboratory to orient the new crown to the teeth in the arch opposing the implant. A dental arch is synonymous with a jaw. There are two arches, the upper arch and the lower arch. The word arch comes from the curved shape of the jaws.

This routine can be somewhat variable and open to the preferences of the individual dentist, but the outcome is the same. Some dentists will use what is known as an "open tray" technique to take the impression, believing that the impression coping will maintain a more accurate position relative to the implant body. This just means that the copings will protrude through the tray used to take the impression and they can be unscrewed and removed with the impression so as not to have to reinsert them afterwards. Everyone develops their own techniques for accomplishing the same thing, and will generally stick with what they know best and works well for them.

I should mention here that the three-piece implant structure that I have described can also be modified if the need arises and according to the preferences of the dentist. The implant body can be made as one piece, with the abutment and the whole thing surgically placed at one time. Alternatively, the whole implant, abutment, and crown can be made as one piece and placed at one time. These options are much less common than the three-piece approach. They allow for the patient to get the final tooth (teeth) in place much sooner, but have fewer options for fixing problems if they should arise down the road. Most dentists are more comfortable with the three-piece design currently in favor, but as materials, imaging techniques, and other advancements in the state of the art continue to evolve, the two- and or one-piece designs may become less risky and more common.

Summary

So now we've talked about the implant body and how it is surgically "implanted" in the jawbone.

These implants then serve to support some sort of an abutment or attachment that can then anchor an individual crown to fill in a space left by a missing tooth or a fixed bridge to replace several consecutively missing teeth.

Finally, they can be used to support an attachment that will anchor a removable denture to replace missing teeth in different parts of the jaw. We've talked about the materials used to construct these implants and the various parts.

The next most common question people have is, of course, about the cost of implants. The answer to cost is complex and varied, so let's get into it.

How Much Do Dental Implants Cost?

The cost of dental implants is highly variable: it depends on the area in which you live, the dentist you go to, your insurance coverage, and the individual characteristics of your own treatment plan. I will give some figures here that I have researched, but these are offered only as a very general ball park estimate of the various costs involved and are not meant to be any actual estimate of anyone's specific treatment cost.

All figures quoted here are given as ranges rather than exact numbers. Again, they are merely general estimates and were gleaned primarily from the following two sources: the *AAID* (*American Academy of Implant Dentistry*) and the *DICG* (*Dental Implant Cost Guide*).

The implant treatment process consists of a number of procedures which are usually separately billed procedures.

Imaging:

The specialized imaging needed for the implant treatment planning can run from $500–$2,500.

The types of images that can be required include single film radiographs of the bone and any remaining teeth in the area of proposed implants. This includes teeth still to be extracted and teeth that will be left (neighboring the proposed implants).

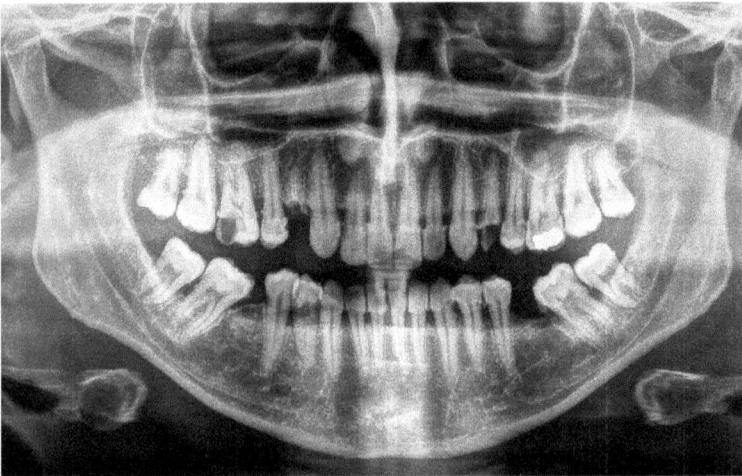

A panographic x-ray of the whole upper and lower jaw is usually required. This will give a much better view of the relationships of bone depth (not thickness) and placement of structures such as the sinus and mandibular nerve and root placements of adjacent teeth.

A CBCT scan will often be used to assess the available bone thickness as well as the desired angle of placement for the implants, among other things.

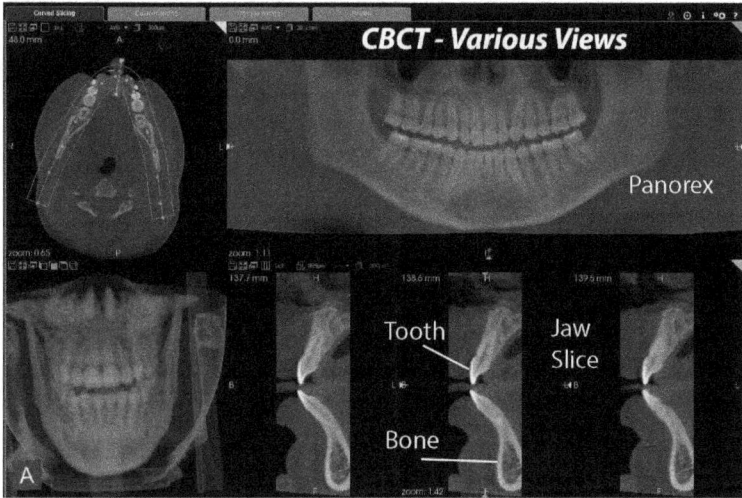

CBCT - Various Views

Extractions:

The cost of extracting teeth (if necessary) is also highly variable and can run from $500–$1,200 per tooth. Tooth extractions can sometimes be done in conjunction with bone augmentation of the extraction socket. The teeth can be whole and vertically oriented (making extraction simpler) or badly broken down (decayed or fractured) and impacted against other structures (making extraction a more complex procedure). There may be only one tooth to extract, several consecutive teeth to extract (adjacent positions in the jaw), or there may be teeth in different parts of the jaw or in both jaws (upper and lower) to extract.

There may be health considerations requiring multiple visits, special medication given, or general anesthesia applied during surgery. Sometimes extra post-op visits will be required to monitor medical complications.

Bone Augmentation:

Bone augmentation costs can be anywhere from $500 in simple cases to $3,500 with complex sinus lift or other procedures.

Bone grafting is a complex subject in itself and beyond the scope of this book. I will just give a basic overview of some of the major types of grafting done classified by materials used, as these can affect the cost of the procedures done. However, the choice of material and procedures required will be made by your professional surgeon, and is not an interactive discussion with you. This is due to many complicated factors involved, not the least of which are the surgeon's own preferences from their past experience.

An autograft is a bone graft where the graft material is obtained from the same person in whom the graft is being placed. This means that bone will be harvested from one site and then placed in another site in the same person. That makes for a more complex surgery due to the necessity of two surgical sites.

An allograft is the use of graft tissue from another human. The bone is usually harvested from a cadaver and preserved, ready to be used when a grafting procedure is done.

A xenograft is a graft using bone from another species (such as bovine).

An alloplastic graft is the use of a synthetic material such as hydroxyapatite.

Each of these materials has different cost factors and different properties, drawbacks, and advantages. Your surgeon can explain the differences in more detail and can tell you why he/she will use a specific modality, but as I mentioned above, the choice is usually not a joint decision but will rest with the surgeon and their expertise.

Surgical Placement:

The implant placement surgery itself can run from $1,000–$3,000. This range is per implant and will vary from geographical region to region as well as depend upon the particular brand or company making the implant parts. The range given here is highly approximate and can vary much more than this, but it gives you a ball park for opening a discussion with your dentist. The manufacturing company is again chosen by the surgeon/dentist team according to the needs of the case and the system they employ for their implants.

Restoration:

The abutment and crown restoration of the implant can run from $800–$3,000. These figures are for single tooth implant procedures and are only broad estimates encompassing a wide range of factors.

The abutments can be a standard abutment purchased from the manufacturer of the implant system being used. They can be custom abutments, sometimes from the manufacturer, sometimes needing to be specifically cast or made by the dental laboratory according to specifications from the restorative dentist. The more customization needed, the higher the cost in general.

The crowns can be a full cast metal crown (usually precious metal—a gold alloy) or can be ceramic (porcelain) or a combination of cast metal (gold-platinum-palladium alloy) with ceramic baked on for esthetic finishing.

If implants are used to support or stabilize a full removable denture, it will usually require four implants (two on each side of the arch). The cost of the attachments that are placed in the implants are relatively similar to the cost of abutments for an implant supported crown. Then the denture will need to be custom made, with the parts inserted inside the denture matching the attachments on the implants for snapping the implants to place. This can increase the cost of the denture from $500–$1,500 on average.

An equally important factor in evaluating the overall cost of an implant treatment plan is the value of implants as compared to the alternatives. None of the traditional restorative options for replacing missing teeth has the degree of comfort and natural feeling that implants do. Implants don't require any alteration of adjacent tooth structure. Implants are currently being reported in the literature as having anywhere from a 95% to 98% success rate, which is higher than any other tooth replacement alternative treatment. There is no more natural looking way to replace a missing tooth in the front of the mouth.

Due to the high success rate and longevity of a typical implant case, the higher cost of initial treatment can be balanced against the greater cost of replacing or repairing alternative treatments such as root canals with dowel posts and crowns, fixed bridges, and removable dentures.

Insurance coverage for implant procedures is growing amongst insurance plans because the success rate has improved over past years. If you are thinking about implants, be sure to check with your insurance company to see how much of the treatment can be covered. Even if the implants themselves are not covered, often some of the surgical procedures may be. Extractions are typically covered in most dental plans. Sometimes bone augmentation procedures and sinus lift procedures are covered under medical plans. The imaging techniques used for dental implants, usually more costly than typical dental x-rays, are sometimes covered by dental or medical insurance.

Summary

So in this chapter we have discussed the various factors involved in the breakdown of costs in an implant case. We discussed the factors that affect the costs of the various procedures involved: imaging, grafting, placement and restoration as well as the extractions that may be needed prior to implant placement.

We discussed some cost ranges as ball park figures to get a general idea of costs involved and a starting point for your own discussions with your dentist. The next thing most people want to know after finding out more about what they are and what costs are involved is whether they can benefit from dental implants in their situation. Let's talk about that next.

What About Me? Am I a Candidate for Dental Implants?

This question really consists of two parts: Can I have dental implants? . . . and Do I want dental implants? As mentioned earlier, I will address the second part of this question at the end of the book. The first part, "Can I have dental implants?" involves a discussion of various factors that would increase the risk of implant failure or risk your ongoing medical health.

Systemic medical conditions impose higher risks of complications from surgical procedures or a higher risk of implant failure. Although very few are absolute contraindications to dental implants, certainly some are more serious than others.

Diseases of the immune system produce high risks of infection that can cause severe complications during surgical procedures as well as ongoing risks of infection around the dental implants. If you have any systemic condition which affects your immune system, a conversation between yourself, your medical doctor and your dental surgeon is mandatory.

Having a compromised immune system is a complication, but not an absolute contraindication for dental implants. Indeed, sometimes the value of improved nutrition provided by having implants that enable the chewing capability required to eat foods with higher fiber content overshadows the increased risks of infections.

If the decision to use implants is made, then certainly before any implant procedures are started, you will have to establish a healthy periodontal condition with regular dental prophylaxis and good home care habits. Any local sites of chronic infection, however slight, should be treated and assessed for ongoing manageability. This includes any periodontal "pockets" (deep crevices between the crest of the gums and the place where the gum attaches to the tooth). Any ongoing marginal inflammation of the gums or carious lesions (cavities) in the teeth need to be addressed.

Your doctor and your dental surgeon will also want to monitor your white blood cell count to make sure your infection fighting capability is optimum for your condition.

Diabetes is a systemic condition affecting the body's ability to regulate blood sugar. It is well known that diabetes patients have increased risks of infection. Infection during the healing phase after surgery is affected, of course, but the ongoing risk of periodontal disease should also be considered. Patients with diabetes should be managing their periodontal health well prior to any dental implant therapy and committed to ongoing rigorous hygiene habits to maintain good oral and periodontal health. Type 2 diabetes is easier to treat and control than type 1. Also patients who have been recently diagnosed have less risk of complications than patients who have had the condition for a longer time.

Since the body's main defense against infection and the main source of tissue nourishment and repair is blood, any systemic conditions affecting blood chemistry should be carefully evaluated prior to planning for dental implants. Conditions which impair the control of bleeding will need evaluation. Medications that prevent clotting will usually need to be stopped for a period of time prior to surgery. If you are prone to excessive bleeding (hemophilia), you may need to have tranexamic acid or epsilon aminocaproic acid prescribed for a period post-operatively to stop excess bleeding.

One systemic condition that has received a lot of public attention with regard to dental treatments is osteoporosis (a systemic condition leading to decreased bone density) and specifically, the medications used to treat osteoporosis (known as bisphosphonates). The common brand names of bisphosphonate medications are Fosamax, Actonel, Boniva, and others like these. Osteoporosis is not automatically a contraindication to dental implant treatment. Implants can be designed to provide more surface area for more bone contact to better anchor it in bone.

The biggest concern with osteoporosis was with the realization that bisphosphonate medications used to treat osteoporosis could also complicate the bone's ability to heal after surgical trauma. Some cases hit the news in which people who were receiving this medication, and then had some dental surgical procedures done, developed osteonecrosis (in which an area of bone dies and needs to be removed). These were serious cases and for a while, anyone taking these medications was afraid to have any dental surgery even though surgeons were taking precautions by conferring with the medical doctors and planning the surgeries with a period of abstinence from the bisphosphonate medication.

Studies have shown that patients on oral doses of these medications have much less risk of surgical complications than patients requiring much heavier intravenous doses. Recent research (*International Journal of Oral and Maxillofacial Implants*, Vol 21: 349) has shown a lowered success rate in patients with osteoporosis, but the difference was less than 2%. If treatment planning is done carefully, taking into account the degree of osteoporosis present, the type of medications prescribed, and the patient's general medical health, people with osteoporosis can be successfully treated with dental implants.

Localized oral health conditions and habits can also influence the success of proposed dental implants. If you have a history of periodontal disease, this should be treated before implants are started. The necessary cleaning and scaling of the teeth, exposed root surfaces, and any possible surgery needed to treat areas of bone loss around teeth that prevent adequate access to tooth brushing and flossing needs to be done first. Then an evaluation of your home care habits must be done to ensure that periodontal health is maintained and the results monitored. It is usually a good idea to consider removal of any remaining teeth that are at high risk due to lack of adequate bone support due to the periodontal disease and include these areas in the dental implant planning.

Bruxism is a habit of "chewing on your teeth" (grinding) or clenching your teeth habitually. There are many factors involved in bruxism, including jaw anatomy, tooth loss or position, and stress, to name a few. Most tooth grinding occurs at night during sleep, while clenching usually happens more during the day (although subconsciously).

Natural teeth are attached to the jawbone with little ligament fibers called periodontal ligaments. This means that the teeth are actually suspended in the bony socket with a ligament "sling." This is important because of the way living bone behaves. Bone normally dissolves when constant pressure is applied to a bone surface. Bone tends to grow when tension is applied to the bone surface. In other words, if you push on the bone it dissolves, if you pull on the bone it grows. This is how orthodontists "move" teeth through the bone. When bands are applied to the teeth, they push on the bone on the side they are moving towards and pull on the bone on the side they are moving away from. The bone dissolves on one side and grows on the other. This has to be done in a slow and controlled fashion. If done too quickly, the dissolution of bone will overwhelm the ability to grow new bone and the teeth will literally move out of the bone.

Implants have no periodontal ligaments. The bone "adheres" to the implant surface directly. Therefore, any forces applied to the implant cause compressive (pressure) forces on the bone. There is no corresponding tension (pulling) force. Bone is able to withstand vertical compressive forces, but will break down quickly with lateral compressive forces. Implants have to be designed and incorporated with the existing teeth so that biting and chewing only causes vertical forces against the implant.

If you have a habit of grinding or clenching, the chances of increasing lateral forces on an implant are multiplied exponentially. The risks of the implant failing (getting loose) goes way up under these conditions. Your dentist will evaluate your "bite pattern" carefully before designing your treatment plan. They will endeavor to limit lateral forces on your implant(s) by balancing your occlusion on the natural teeth as well as evaluating the final implant restoration(s) to make sure the bite patterns are not harmful to the new implant(s). Even without bruxism, it is always recommended that patients be fitted for an occlusal guard (i.e., night guard, bite plate) to minimize the risk of excess lateral forces on the implant.

Smoking is another habit that can cause increased risk of implant failure. The hot gases can burn the oral cavity and damage salivary glands. Nicotine in smoke reduces blood flow to the soft tissues, which can affect the immune response and slow the healing process. At the same time, smoking promotes the growth of disease-causing oral bacteria. Smoking obviously has many adverse effects to general health as well, but these specific local effects can reduce the chances of success with your implants. The literature shows mixed results, but it is generally agreed that the success rate in smokers versus non-smokers is much reduced, possibly by half.

This does not mean that smokers can't have implants, but that they should take every care to reduce any other risk factors that can be managed and should be monitored closely during healing and ongoing afterward. If you are a smoker and need implants, it would be best if you quit smoking before treatment. I know this is not an easy thing; my own father tried to quit smoking at least three times that I know of and only succeeded finally after a quadruple bypass surgery, but the overall health benefits to quitting, as well as the benefit to your planned implant treatment, makes the attempt well worth it.

Anatomical considerations can also influence the dental implant process. These are not considered contraindications but I include them here as part of the question "Can I Get Implants?" because they have to be included in the treatment planning process and do affect the overall time and expense that you are looking at.

The first of these is the position of the maxillary sinus cavity relative to the desired implant placement site. If there is not enough bone between the crest of the jaw ridge and the floor of the sinus, a "sinus lift" procedure is necessary, along with some addition of bone graft material, to provide room to place the implant. This procedure usually adds 4-8 months onto the dental implant process, as this has to heal and the bone grafting material integrate with the bone before placing the implants.

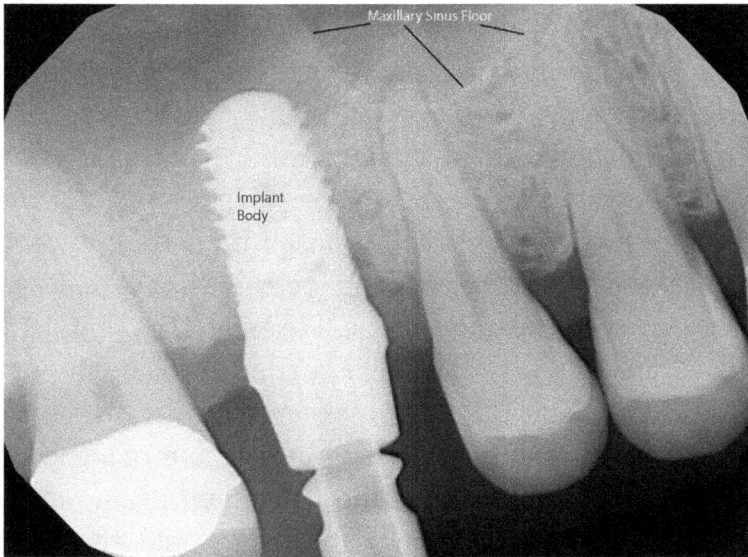

Maxillary Sinus Floor

Implant Body

*Shows relative position of implant to floor of sinus
(This could be the natural contour of sinus floor or
sinus lift may have been done here)*

The second is the mandibular canal, carrying the mandibular nerve through the lower jaw. The position of the nerve canal relative to the crest of the ridge is important again to determine if enough depth of bone exists in the area of the proposed implant(s) for their placement. Sometimes these areas will also need to be augmented with grafting materials to provide adequate depth of bone for the implant(s). That can also add an additional 4-8 months to the overall treatment plan.

The lower jaw also presents another consideration. The jawbone itself is usually angled outward towards the lower edge of the jaw. The jaw can be very thin from the outer to inner surface, so that even with adequate depth from crest to nerve canal, there is not enough bone around the proposed implant to anchor it. If the surrounding bone is too thin, it will dissolve during the healing phase, leaving the implant inadequately supported. The angle of the bone may make it difficult to position an implant with the long axis of the implant parallel to the long axis of adjacent teeth. If the jaw ridge is too thin, then again, some bone augmentation will be necessary and the time allotted for completion of the treatment plan increased.

Another anatomical consideration is the vertical distance between the jaws at rest. At rest means you are not actively trying to open your mouth, nor are you biting down. Your dentist will measure this and determine if there is enough vertical space to place an implant, an abutment, and a crown. If the implants are to be used to stabilize a full or partial removable denture, there has to be enough vertical space to place the implant, the attachments, and the denture with the mating parts of the attachments built into it.

If the vertical space is too small to accommodate these parts of an implant case, then there are ways to increase the vertical dimension, but they will significantly increase the time and cost of the overall treatment plan. If the vertical space is too small, it usually indicates that the vertical space has collapsed due to tooth wear or tooth loss over time. The risks to the jaw joints of leaving the vertical space collapsed involves development of TMJ or TMD (temporo-mandibular joint syndrome or temporo-mandibular dysfunction). This could be a very painful and difficult condition to treat in advanced stages. If you can correct the problem, your risk of later discomfort is much less.

These anatomical variations are not factors that prevent implant treatment but can, as mentioned, affect the overall time and cost as well as require going through some extra surgical procedures to provide optimal conditions for success. I would state here that the augmentation procedures mentioned above are different from bone grafting materials being added to the existing tooth socket at the time of the extraction of a tooth. The bone augmentation I have discussed in relation to added cost and time involved means the augmentation of bone where bone was deficient due to previous tooth loss or anatomical variation. When teeth are extracted immediately prior to implant therapy, the space vacated by the tooth root can also be augmented (filled).This is done to aid in the healing of the socket with minimal bone loss during the healing and does not necessarily add time to the implant treatment plan. The cost for this is also usually minimal, but well worth it.

Summary

In this chapter we discussed the various conditions that would either prevent or increase your risk of complications with dental implants. I broke these down into systemic medical conditions, localized oral health conditions and habits, and anatomical considerations.

Most of the conditions I have discussed have varying degrees of severity or advancement in any particular case. In some cases, dental implants can be planned and executed with careful consideration of the factors involved. In other cases, it may be best to consider an alternative to the implants. This is where you and your dentist can (in conjunction with your medical doctor, in some cases) discuss your options and make appropriate decisions.

This was a generalized discussion of some of the more common considerations and gives you enough information to have and understand a discussion with your dentist about your own situation. This book is not meant to substitute for a discussion with your dentist nor to be offered as an argument for any dentist's opinion about your treatment. The dentist doing an exam has access to all the pertinent facts regarding your case and their opinion should be respected above all. I offer this book and the information provided here to enable you to be more prepared to ask meaningful questions and understand the answers your dentist provides.

Immediately following the question about their own candidacy for dental implants, most people will want to know if the dental implant procedures and dental implants themselves are safe. That's an excellent question. Let's talk about that.

Are Dental Implants Safe? How Long Do They Last?

These two questions are asked frequently and usually separately, but are closely related. Sometimes when people ask the first question about safety, it's really just another way of wording the second question about longevity. However, there are other implications about the safety question that I'll talk about here.

Surgical Factors

The term "surgery" itself carries a connotation for people that often induces fear of pain and/or complications. The placement of an implant is usually easier (safer) than the extraction that created the need for the implant. Once the bone site is ready for implant placement, the procedure involves drilling a small hole through the overlying gum tissue and into the bone. This may sound harsh or scary, but of all the people I have worked with, almost everyone has reported that the actual surgery was much easier than they expected. The procedure doesn't take long (usually less time than an extraction) and local anesthesia makes it quite painless. They also usually report very little, if any, post-operative pain. In some cases, a surgeon will elect to make an incision to pull the gum tissue back out of the way and suture it back over the implant site afterwards, but this makes little difference in the reports that patients give of their experience.

Additional surgical procedures (also called adjunctive procedures), such as sinus lift or ridge augmentation, can be longer in duration, but are usually relatively safe from complications compared to extraction of teeth. The main risk of sinus lift surgery is tearing the sinus membrane. If this occurs, a repair will be attempted. If repair can't be completed at the time, the surgeon may have to stop and close it up, wait for the tear to heal, and then complete the sinus lift later. This can involve more time and post-operative pain than usual. There are newer techniques available to do this surgery with less risk of tearing the sinus membrane, and most surgeons performing this procedure are using the latest techniques available.

There are a number of techniques used for increasing the vertical dimension of a jaw ridge (different from the vertical dimension of space between the jaws discussed in the last chapter) with bone augmentation. Discussion of these is rather technical and not really necessary for you to know about. Just know that if this is needed in your case, the surgeon will be using whatever technique he or she is most comfortable with and thinks will provide the best result. Complications that would increase the time and/or cost of your treatment are possible with any of these techniques, and you should be made aware of the possibilities ahead of time.

In spite of the possibility of complications with any surgery, more and more people are getting dental implants place every year. The majority of cases go ahead without significant complications and are completed quite successfully.

Non-Surgical Factors

The materials used for implants are biocompatible and involve little risk of rejection by the body, but it is a slight possibility. In some cases, if an implant is placed too close to a nerve, pain and/or numbness can result. This can be either temporary or permanent. This same risk is true of any tooth extraction.

If the implants are placed in bone that is not dense enough or healthy enough, the implant may lose bone around it during the first year and eventually become loose. If the implant is overloaded, meaning the biting forces apply too much pressure (especially lateral pressure), the implant can also become loose. After implant placements, patients are usually fitted with an occlusal guard to minimize risks of failure due to occlusal stress. If an implant becomes loose, it will need to be removed and either replaced or an alternative treatment used.

The screw holding the abutment to the implant may become loose over time. This usually just involves removing the crown, re-tightening the screw, and then re-cementing the crown. This is not an uncommon occurrence. The cement used to "fix" the crown to the abutment is specially made for implant crowns. It is somewhat softer than traditional crown and bridge cements and not a bonded cement. It is made this way so that the crown can be removed without damaging the underlying abutment, so the screw may be tightened and the crown re-cemented. The crown itself may get loose, and this just means it needs to be re-cemented. This might happen more often with an implant crown because of the nature of the specialized cement mentioned above.

Longevity of an implant case is quite good compared to other methods of tooth replacement. It was mentioned already that implants have, according to most literature reports today, a 95-98% success rate. This means that after five years, the implants are still stable and functioning with adequate bone support. Some studies have reported a 90% success rate over ten years. Most studies have shown that crowns and bridges usually last 8-10 years before needing to be replaced or the supporting tooth removed. It is generally agreed upon in the profession that implants last much longer than fixed bridges. One very big reason for this difference is that implants have no risk of underlying tooth decay. Periodontally, they have the same risks of infection as natural teeth. This means that crowns or bridges can fail for all the same reasons that implants would, but they also have the risk of decay or fracture of the supporting tooth under the crown or bridge prosthesis.

One of the main reasons that patients who are deciding between implants and an alternative treatment for their missing teeth choose an alternative method is the initial cost and time investment for implants. It should be pointed out that these alternative methods will usually require some replacement in a much shorter time than an implant. So the question of longevity is an important one. The initial investment (both money and time) for implants will most likely be less than the overall investment required for an alternative treatment in the long run.

Imaging Factors

A word should be said here about the imaging techniques available to dentists today with regard to the safety and longevity of dental implants. As you probably gathered from the discussion above, many of the risks of dental implant placement involve placing the implant in the wrong place. Knowing where an implant can be successfully placed and where some augmentation will be needed is a large part of the battle to create a successful implant case.

When dental implants were in their early years of development, the success rates were rather poor because dentists could only use conventional x-rays and indirect physical measurements to assess the location and thickness of bone. At best, x-rays give only give a two-dimensional picture of the bone in any area. With early implants, the jaw was often perforated, the mandibular nerve encroached upon, or the maxillary sinus perforated. Implants were placed too close to each other or too close to an adjacent tooth root.

These problems have been largely solved by the advent of cone beam computed tomography (CBCT). This is a specialized version of computed axial tomography (CAT scan), which was developed in the 1970's and used largely for medical purposes. CBCT was first introduced in Europe in 1996 and in the U.S. in 2001.

CBCT involves using a moving head shooting divergent x-rays through a target area and computing an image that represents a 3D image of the target area. Although the absolute density of the bone imaged with this technique can't be accurately assessed, the location, thickness, and relative density can be visually assessed very easily. This is an enormous aid in placing dental implants confidently. Using this type of image, along with a physical model of the jaw with a surgical template, makes implant placement much more accurate than ever before.

A surgical template is a plastic device made on the stone model of your teeth and jaws. It is made with data obtained from 3D images as well as visual assessment of existing teeth. It has been drilled with holes that are parallel to the desired path of insertion of the implant and wide enough to admit the drill used to prepare and place the implant, thus directing the drill without guess work. Such a template is not always required, but can be extremely useful in some circumstances.

Summary

We have just discussed the surgical, non-surgical, and imaging factors that combine to make implants not only safe, but arguably the longest lasting restorative option for replacement of missing teeth.

We talked a little about the actual surgical process of placing an implant in the bone. We talked about the most common adjunctive surgical procedures that are called for in some cases.

We talked about the use of an occlusal guard after treatment to minimize chewing and grinding stresses and the specialized implant cement used to facilitate repair of minor problems (such as a loose abutment screw). The use of a surgical template to guide the implant placement was discussed.

Finally we talked about the improved imaging techniques available today and how they greatly improve the safety of the implant process.

The next question most people ask is, "OK, I understand how safe they are, but how much will it hurt?"

How Painful Is the Process?

Questions about pain are natural. Nobody wants to feel pain. These questions are also difficult to give a simple answer to because there is no simple answer. Pain is a very subjective experience. Two people can go through the same experience and one will say it was very painful and the other will say it hardly hurt at all.

However, there are some general things that can be said about the implant process with respect to the expectation of pain. All surgeries are invasive, meaning they involve cutting into or drilling into living tissue. The state of local and general anesthesia today makes most surgical procedures painless during the process. So what most people are asking is: will it hurt afterwards?

Post-operative pain depends largely on the degree of tissue invasion that is necessary. If a simple, one tooth implant is placed without any need for bone augmentation or sinus lift surgery and no soft tissue flap is needed, then generally there is very little post-operative pain involved. A soft tissue flap is when the surgeon needs to make an incision in the gum tissue and pull it out of the way to directly expose the bone. If a flap process is done for visibility or access, rather than for the need to do some bone augmentation or sinus surgery, there is usually a little more post-operative pain, but still generally tolerable with either over-the-counter pain relievers or a mild dose of prescription pain medication.

Post-operative pain is generally more profound when adjunctive surgeries have to be done to prepare the implant site. These include the bone augmentation and sinus lift procedures discussed in the last chapter as well as other procedures that are sometimes required that are outside the scope of this book. That is because these procedures require a more invasive technique and manipulation of gum and bone tissue, and usually take longer and have more bleeding. This, again, is subjective, with some people experiencing more pain and some hardly any.

Post-operative pain is managed with pain medication, either prescription or non-prescription. Non-prescription (over-the-counter or OTC) medications include both non-steroidal anti-inflammatory drugs (NSAIDS) and other analgesics (acetaminophen being most common). Examples of brand names for this class of pain relievers are:

NSAID:

   Aspirin
      Anacin
      Bayer

Bufferin
Excedrin (actually a combination of
acetaminophen, aspirin and caffeine)
Ibuprofen
Advil
Motrin
Nuprin
Naproxen
Aleve
Naprosyn

Not NSAID:

Acetaminophen (not anti-inflammatory—
reduces pain by elevating pain threshold)
Tylenol
Paracetamol

When something stronger than over-the-counter (OTC) pain relievers are called for, it will usually be a narcotic analgesic (codeine or hydrocodone or oxycodone) combined with acetaminophen (Vicodin, Norco, Percocet) or with an NSAID (Vicoprofen, Ibudone).

Whenever a drug is prescribed by your dentist for pain relief, pay attention to their directions and read the label carefully; refresh yourself on the correct dosage and timing to ensure it is taken as directed for best results and least danger of overdose. If you think your pain level requires more medication or stronger medication, call your dentist and discuss what you are feeling with them. It is important that your dentist and surgeon are made aware of any medications you have been prescribed for other conditions, so drug harmful drug interactions can be avoided.

Once the implants have integrated with the bone and are now stable enough to have the abutment and crown (or attachments and dentures) placed on them, the process is relatively simple, especially from your point of view.

The implant body has had a screw with a large head (sometimes called a healing cap) placed hold the gum tissue position. The dentist unscrews the healing cap, places an impression coping (also with a screw), takes the impression, removes the coping, and replaces the healing cap. This is all painless and quite fast. No anesthetic is usually required. The impression is sent to the laboratory to make the abutment and crown, and some time later (usually a couple of weeks), you return to the dentist for the placement of the final crown. This is also relatively quick and without anesthetic, as all that is required is unscrewing and screwing of the parts attached to the implant body, followed by cementation of crown(s) or bridge.

The process is longer if a denture is involved, as the denture requires more impressions and measurement visits than crowns, but in terms of pain, the process is the same in that nothing painful is involved in these visits. After delivery of a denture, sore spots may need adjusting to "fine tune" the fit of the denture where they still sit on the gum tissue over the jawbone. Usually, these dentures require far less adjustment and have far fewer sore spots than traditional dentures because the main support for the dentures is the implant, not the soft tissue.

Summary

We have seen in this chapter that "pain," relative to dental implants, usually means post-operative pain after the surgical portion of the treatment. The restorative phase is generally very easy for patients, involving very little or no pain and generally requiring no local anesthetic.

The post-operative pain involved can vary with the amount and degree of surgery required for a particular situation. As always, every person also has their own pain threshold. What might be relatively painful for one person may be quite pain-free for another.

There are a number of options for medically treating the post-operative pain that does occur, and I have discussed some of the more popular options above.

So, if dental implants are so safe, long lasting, and relatively pain-free, what are the downsides? Let's explore the answer to that question in the next chapter.

What Are the Downsides of Dental Implants?

For most people, there are several drawbacks to dental implants that share center stage in their considerations. *The first is the cost* of the procedures involved. This can be especially true if their treatment plan calls for the extra surgeries that I discussed earlier.

The cost of getting implants can definitely be high compared to alternative treatments, and this is something that every person needs to decide for themselves. Most people get an estimate of the cost involved and then decide, based on just the numbers, whether they can afford the implants or not. Many people are already convinced that implants are beyond their means before they even have the estimate.

I think that it is important, if you are considering implants, to consider the value of the implants before, or at least along with, the costs. Many people don't realize the full extent of benefits provided by implants. Because they are inserted in the bone, they tend to preserve the jawbone, even without the periodontal ligaments that natural teeth have.

They are also more hygienic than bridges or partial dentures because they can be flossed as well as brushed just like natural teeth. Implants are not subject to dental decay, one of the main causes for failure of crowns and fixed bridges. If an implant integrates well with the bone and is maintained well by follow-up visits to the dentist and good home care habits, implants can often be expected to long outlast traditional restorative options like crowns, bridges, and partial dentures.

If you think about the cost of replacing bridges and partial dentures as being part of their cost versus the longevity of dental implants, the cost factor starts to lean much more in favor of dental implants, in spite of the initial higher cost.

The *second drawback that discourages many people is the time* involved in the treatment. A full course of treatment for dental implants can range from 6 months to well over a year, depending on adjunctive procedures required, number of implants, patient health, and other factors.

This is again a personal decision that should be considered after all the facts are gathered. Sometimes people have suffered tooth loss for a long time prior to considering implants. In these cases, time is not usually so important psychologically. However, if someone is having existing teeth extracted in conjunction with proposed implants, or have only recently lost the teeth in question, they are often appalled at the idea that they won't get teeth back in the spaces for 6 months or more. This becomes most important with front teeth, where the missing teeth are visibly noticeable or when many teeth are missing and people are worried about their nutritional needs if they can't chew properly.

The reality is that when these situations exist, the dentist will include a temporary denture, often called a stayplate, in the treatment plan to provide an esthetic solution for front teeth and a functional solution for back teeth. These temporary dentures are not as secure as the final restorations nor usually as esthetic, but they are much better than doing without the teeth altogether.

These temporary dentures do involve an added cost, but most patients consider them well worth the cost. The cost of a temporary denture usually is a small fraction of the overall treatment cost, and range from $200–$600 on average. Most dentists will try to keep this cost down because they understand that the overall treatment plan is already high enough to become a perceived barrier for many people. Some dentists will charge only their laboratory cost, while others will discount the fee to some extent.

This is an individual decision by the dentist; they have to consider their laboratory costs, chair time for impressions and delivery, and then additional chair time for adjustments. You should understand that if a dentist quotes a fee for this part of the treatment, he or she has already considered all these factors and it is not worth trying to bargain for a "deal." If you trust your dentist, trust that they are doing their best to be fair and to give you more value than cost. If you don't trust your dentist, get another dentist.

The other aspect of the time factor is personal health. Sometimes people of advanced age do not feel like they want to put themselves through a time-consuming treatment plan. This is a valid decision and should be respected. The same can be true if people have compromising health issues. Their health issues may not be absolute contraindications to dental implants, but may be psychologically something they just don't want to go through.

The third drawback to dental implants is risk of failure. Even though the success rate for implants is statistically very high, the truth is that implants, like anything else, sometimes fail. What it means for an implant to fail is one of two things. A complete failure means the implant must be removed and either attempted again or an alternative treatment considered. A partial failure means some part of the implant construction has failed and requires a repair.

Complete failures usually involve loosening of the implant body itself. Either the integration with the bone was never fully realized, or forces on the implant after placement of the abutment and crown portion have caused the breakdown of that integration. If the body rejects the implant, rare but possible, then integration with the bone is never achieved and the implant becomes loose even before the restorative phase (when the abutment and crown portions of the implant would be placed). If the implant does integrate well and the next phase of the implant restoration is completed, then biting and chewing can cause lateral displacement forces on the implant. This can cause breakdown of the bone attachment and the implant will loosen.

A third cause of loss of bone attachment and loosening of an implant is perioimplantitis. Just as periodontitis causes breakdown of the periodontal ligaments holding teeth to the bone, perioimplantitis causes breakdown of the integration of bone to implant. Plaque must be removed from around implant restorations just as religiously as it is removed from natural teeth to preserve the health of the structures (gum and bone tissue) supporting the implant.

Good oral hygiene habits have to be maintained and regular recall visits to your dentist for regular cleanings are a must. In addition, the bone and gum tissue health around the implant body and abutment need to be regularly assessed to detect, early on, any breakdown occurring due to infection, inflammation, or occlusal (biting) stresses.

The fourth drawback to dental implants for some people is the surgery itself. For whatever reason, some people just do not like to have any surgery done regardless of any benefits obtainable. These are people who usually would only consent to a surgical procedure if it were necessary to sustain their life or if the problem impacts their quality of life enough to justify overcoming their resistance to surgery. Reasons for this can be very complex and very deep, and usually have nothing to do with dentistry and even less to do with the individual dentist. I would venture to guess that if you are reading this book, this is not you. In my experience, people who feel this way about surgery don't search out more information about surgical procedures—they just avoid them.

Most people, however, are not eager to have surgical procedures and will research their risks, benefits, and options carefully. This is normal and admirable. You are the people for whom I am writing this book.

Having said this, however, there is the possibility that for some people who want dental implants and wouldn't mind the basic implant surgery, their treatment plans involve enough adjunctive surgery for bone augmentation and/or sinus lift that they will decline or hold off on the dental implant treatment. It is important to honestly evaluate your own comfort level with any proposed treatment plan and to discuss this with your dentist ahead of time. As a dentist, the last thing I want to do is convince someone to go ahead with a treatment if they really don't want it. In the long run, this will cause me problems as well as be a disservice to the patient.

Sometimes people make decisions based on factors that have nothing to do with dentistry or that they do not feel comfortable talking about with the dentist or the dental staff. This is fine, but it is important that you are clear with your dentist about what you do or don't want to have done (whether you fully discuss your reasons or not). If you have a good dentist (and I'm talking about most dentists), they will respect your decisions as long as they have been able to give you all the information you need to make an informed decision.

Summary

The drawbacks to dental implants usually involve people's reaction to:

Money
Time
Risk of failure
Aversion to surgery

Your position with respect to each of these drawbacks should be balanced against the benefits you could experience from having implants, and then decide what works for you. Make sure you are clear with your dentist about what you want. If you can, explain your own reasons. This will help your dentist adjust your treatment plan to give you your best options.

Many times parents or people in their later years will ask about dental implants with respect to age. Let's look at this next.

Am I Too Old or Too Young for Dental Implants?

This is of course actually two questions, but closely related. The first question, "Am I too old?" is more often stated as a declaration than a question: "I'm too old to be getting implants." The second question is usually asked by a parent rather than the patient: "Is my (son/daughter) too young for dental implants?"

The youth question first.

Although it is not common for children to be considered candidates for implants, there are sometimes cases of congenitally missing teeth which will eventually need to be restored in some way. Because the jawbone is still in development, however, implants, as well as fixed crowns or bridges, are not recommended for anyone under 18 or 19 years of age. Because implants, unlike natural teeth, have no periodontal ligaments, they will not move through the bone as the jaw develops. Therefore, if placed before development is completed, an implant's final position could be out of alignment horizontally and/or vertically from its desired position. Because of the lack of periodontal ligaments, an implant's position cannot be corrected orthodontically; the position can only be corrected surgically by removal and replacement.

The dentist will usually advise some form of space maintainer for your child until they reach an appropriate age for implants (or their alternatives). However, with children, it will often make more sense to use orthodontic movement of the existing permanent teeth to close a gap left by a tooth lost or congenitally missing. There are many variations on this theme and I will not attempt to address them here. That would be more of a discussion about orthodontics and is not in the scope of this book. However, you should be aware of the possible options involving tooth movement as an alternative for tooth replacement.

The other question: "Am I too old for dental implants?"

This is actually the wrong question. A better question is: "Am I healthy enough for implants?" Age is not by itself a contraindication for dental implants nor the surgery they entail. If a person is healthy and vital at any age, they are usually able to have dental implants done. If health is compromised, then a consultation between the patient, the dentist and the medical doctor treating the compromising conditions may be required. The proposed benefits of the dental implants for the particular patient need to be weighed against the increased risks involved with their condition.

Equally, a patient of advanced age with compromising health issues should be evaluated with regard to their willingness to go through the treatment regardless of the benefits proposed, as I mentioned in the last chapter. Just because something can be done doesn't mean it should be.

It is sometimes a question of placing some implants to anchor a denture so that the patient's nutrition improves. The benefit here is obviously an important consideration as any compromising condition will respond better with good nutrition. In this case, every effort should be made to overcome any contraindicating factors and to help the patient realize the importance of the treatment.

Summary

Children should be old enough that their jaws have reached final development before placing implants. This is generally between 18-20 years of age.

It is important with children to consider the possibilities of orthodontic treatment as an alternative to dental implants.

Old age is not itself a contraindication to dental implants. The more important consideration is your relative health. Here again, benefits versus risk should be carefully evaluated.

If you decide not to go with dental implants, then what? What are the alternatives? In the next chapter,

I explore the alternative treatments and their risks versus benefits.

What Are My Alternatives to Dental Implants?

Let's recap for a moment what dental implants are used for. Dental implants are used to replace the roots of missing teeth. These artificial roots can be used to support a single crown for a single missing tooth. They can be used as supports for a fixed bridge to replace several missing teeth. They can be used to support attachments which can act as anchors for a removable partial or full denture.

So, before we had dental implants, what were the alternatives for replacing missing teeth? A single missing tooth has always been the easiest situation for replacement. We could drill on the two teeth on either side of the space where a single tooth was missing and use cement to anchor a fixed bridge to these "prepared" teeth. This is known as a 3-unit bridge and has been around as an alternative for many years.

Fixed bridges could be all gold or have a gold-platinum-palladium alloy base with porcelain baked on to give it a tooth-like appearance. In order to do this, the adjacent teeth had to be assessed as to whether they were strong enough to support a bridge. The process takes about two weeks to complete unless the dentist uses an in-house laboratory, in which case it can be done much faster, often making this option more attractive to people who don't like the long treatment time required for implants.

The strength being assessed was basically of two types, both necessary for long-term survival of the prosthesis. The structure of the visible part of the tooth had to have enough integrity to support the bridge by itself, or it had to be strengthened by some type of build-up material if the tooth structure was severely compromised by decay or tooth fracture.

Quite often when a tooth was missing, the adjacent teeth had already been treated in the past, sometimes multiple times, with fillings. These fillings could often comprise the majority of what was left of the visible tooth. Older filling materials were of a metal called silver amalgam, and these fillings were usually not done with any bonding technology. Most fillings eventually "leak," meaning decay would find its way underneath. If these teeth were to be the support for a new fixed bridge, any possibility of underlying decay needed to be found and fixed. Most old fillings, therefore, had to be fully removed and the tooth structure rebuilt.

This is all still true. Now we can rebuild a tooth with composite resin materials and bonding technology (which is far superior and stronger than the older pin retained silver amalgams), but there is a limit to how much tooth structure can be replaced, even with bonding, and still have something strong enough to predictably retain a fixed bridge for any length of time without breaking.

Our next option, if too much tooth structure was missing to rely on bonding alone, is to remove the nerve from the tooth (if indeed it still has viable nerve tissue), fill the root space with an inert material to prevent bacteria from causing further decay or infection (root canal), and then insert a stainless steel or cast gold dowel post part way into the now non-vital (dead) tooth and bond it to the tooth. The cement used to secure the post into the canal should be a bonded cement as well. This unites the whole post-buildup as a unit with the remaining tooth root. The hope is to add some strength to the buildup process with the post. The problems with this include possibility of infection into the root or fracture of the root from stresses on the bridge translating to the post.

The second type of "strength" we need for a bridge abutment tooth is periodontal strength. The bone holding the tooth in the jaw must be sufficiently strong and healthy (just like we discussed for implants). Unfortunately, periodontally compromised teeth with loss of bone support also have a compromised root structure (where the bone has been lost). There is a natural layer on healthy roots called cementum, which is responsible for maintaining periodontal ligaments. I explained previously how periodontal ligaments were so important for maintaining healthy bone and for the ability of teeth to move within bone successfully. It is also the way that bone and teeth bond and work together. When this layer and the ligaments are gone, it is extremely difficult to do any kind of bone augmentation without removing the rest of the tooth. The more bone has been lost around a given tooth, the more likely the eventual failure of a bridge being supported by that tooth.

In spite of these obstacles to the success of fixed bridges, they have been a mainstay of dental treatment for many years and do serve a valuable function. Due to the compromise of tooth structure needed to place them (or use of already compromised tooth structure) however, dental implants are increasingly recommended for replacing even single missing teeth.

If the single missing tooth is the last one in the back of the jaw, a fixed bridge is not possible in the traditional way because there is no anchor tooth behind the space. A fixed cantilever bridge can be done, anchoring the replacement to the tooth or two teeth in front of the space. The stress on these anchor teeth for a cantilever approach is much greater than that of a traditional bridge, and most dentists will use this approach very sparingly and only with warnings of the likelihood of early failure, possibly not only of the bridge itself but loss of one or more anchor teeth in the process.

With no posterior (back) anchor for a fixed bridge, the only other option for replacement of a missing tooth or teeth (without considering implants) is a removable denture option. Removable dentures rely on a chrome-cobalt cast framework to "grab," or clasp, some of the remaining natural teeth (or teeth with crowns on them) and have plastic teeth set in acrylic to replace the missing teeth. This type of restoration is generally the least expensive of the tooth replacement options and takes anywhere from a couple of weeks to a month to make.

If there are a larger number of missing teeth and they are missing from multiple areas in the jaw, the expense of treating all of the spaces with implants can be a problem due to financial considerations. This can make the partial denture the only viable option. It is worth noting that implants can still be considered at a later date if a person's financial situation changes.

Removable dentures can be either partial (some natural teeth remain), as in the above paragraph, or full (no remaining teeth), in which case there would be only the teeth embedded in an acrylic base plate.

The drawbacks to partial dentures are many. They are much harder to wear as they can be quite uncomfortable and take a lot of getting used to. The framework takes up room in the mouth, affects the taste of food, collects food underneath, and causes a lot of stress on both the teeth it clasps to and the soft tissues it rests on.

Both partial and full dentures can cause sores on the gums and usually need several post-delivery adjustments to "fine tune" the fit. Then comes a period of wearing the denture to get used to the way it feels. Dentures are more easily broken than fixed bridges. This applies to both the metal framework of a partial denture and the plastic part of either a partial or full denture.

One drawback to removable appliances that doesn't exist for fixed prosthetics is what happens when you take them out. They can be lost fairly easily. Some people have taken them out for cleaning in a motel room, wrapped them in tissue paper overnight, and then forgotten them when they left in the morning.

One story I heard from a patient has to be told here. This person had a lower partial denture he had worn for a number of years. He came in one day and said he needed a new lower partial. I asked what the problem was with the old one, so I could make a new one that solved the problem. At first he didn't want to talk about it, but after some prompting, he finally told me: "It got run over by my car." I knew this person well and knew he understood my sense of humor, so I said, "Gee, I hope you weren't wearing it at the time." True story—I swear!

The last alternative to dental implants is no treatment. Sometimes people who lose a tooth or even multiple teeth elect not to do anything and just learn to function with the remaining teeth as best they can. This is not an option I feel good about and don't recommend, but it's not my job to make the decision. It's my job to give you all the information you need to make a good informed decision based on your own priorities.

Like any of the treatment alternatives discussed above, including dental implants, not doing anything has benefits, risks, and alternatives. We've already discussed the alternatives. The benefits are not having to spend any time or money on treatment.

The risks are not so apparent, but can be significant. Natural teeth are "living" in bone. Bone itself is living. When teeth are removed for whatever reason, a balance is disturbed. The forces of chewing and growing and speaking and grinding or clenching all go on. Bacteria still exist in the mouth. Everything goes on, except now there are fewer teeth to absorb these events.

The remaining teeth that are now absorbing more than their share of normal stresses tend to break down faster. This includes enamel wear, tooth fracture, and bone loss. Eventually the "easy way" (no treatment) doesn't seem so easy.

If one tooth is gone, the other teeth may, and often do, drift into the space left. This affects the way they interact with the teeth in the opposing arch. This also affects the jaw joints and, over time, can affect the joints quite a lot, especially if there are any grinding or clenching habits going on. The uneven stresses on the teeth that have moved can lead to nerve death within the tooth, leading to root canal treatment or further tooth loss.

The jaw joint can wear unnaturally, causing degeneration of the cartilage disc cushioning the jaw from the skull. This can lead to arthritis of the jaw joint or bone on bone rubbing of the jaw and skull bones, stretching of the ligaments holding the cartilage in place, etc. All of these and more make up what has come to be called TMD or TMJ, meaning dysfunction of the temporo-mandibular joint. This can involve anything from distracting clicking or popping noises to occasional pains to constant severe aching. Each stage of this syndrome gets progressively harder to treat.

Not everyone who loses a tooth and does nothing will experience these issues, but you should be aware that they do happen and many people do suffer these symptoms. If you don't treat a problem, you are rolling the dice on the likelihood of more severe problems later on.

All of the above alternatives to dental implants include one other significant drawback. The bone in the area of the missing tooth will gradually continue to resorb (dissolve) and make the jaw weaker over time, as well as provide less support for any nearby remaining teeth.

Summary

In this chapter we have seen that there are alternatives to replacing missing teeth with dental implants. Teeth can be replaced with fixed bridges (crowns cemented to the teeth adjacent to the space of the missing tooth) or removable partial or full dentures.

These alternatives have been around much longer than implants. They are generally less expensive than implants and can be delivered in much less time.

The drawbacks to the fixed bridge option involve the compromise of strength to adjacent teeth by preparing them for crowns or the need to use already compromised teeth as the support for the bridge. The possibility of decay or fracture of the supporting teeth leading to the need for a longer bridge, or now having to move to a partial denture, is a risk and an eventual probability.

Dentures, both partial and full, can replace many missing teeth or teeth missing in multiple parts of the jaws. They can be done faster than implants and are the least costly (initially) of the replacement options.

The drawbacks to dentures involve the stress on supporting teeth or tissues. Sores and fitting problems are common. Comfort is never the same as implant-supported restorations or fixed bridges. Dentures can break more easily.

Each treatment assumes a number of risks developing over time. All alternatives to dental implants will involve more gradual loss of bone and jaw integrity over time, whereas dental implants can preserve bone.

It's time to address my thoughts on the question I can't answer for you. When you ask yourself, "Do I Want Dental Implants?" consider this:

Do I Want Dental Implants?

You have now learned what dental implants are and how they are done. You have read some information about the success rates of implants and how they compare with alternative treatments. You've read some information about the cost of implants and some of the possible adjunctive treatments that may have to be done, depending on your jawbone, remaining teeth, state of health, etc. You know something about the post-operative pain level you might expect and what can be done about it, as well as the risks and benefits of implants versus the alternatives. Now there is just one question left for you to ask yourself: "Do I want dental implants?"

It is a good thing to gather as much information as you can before making decisions about anything and to then evaluate the pros and cons of any course of action. After reading this book, you should be in a better position to have a meaningful discussion with your dentist about your particular situation and take part in your own treatment plan. You should be able to understand what your dentist is talking about and ask questions that are relevant using the information from this book.

However, what I think sometimes gets lost by both patients and dentists is the emotional component of any decision, especially decisions about your body and personal health and appearance. You might hear all the reasons why implants would be a terrific benefit to you and still not really want to go through the process for many reasons that are not necessarily apparent or easy to discuss. That does not make them invalid. If something deep down inside you is saying "I don't want to do this," you should probably listen to that. There may be something you still need to know before you can really feel that you want the treatment (or you may not ever want it).

I have had patients who decided to have implants because it sounded like a beneficial thing and/or the latest best thing. Some of them didn't really want the treatment. Perhaps they were influenced by me or by family members or even just ignored their own feelings. Unfortunately, once it has been done, the die is cast, so to speak. In talking with them later, sometimes much later when another implant is contemplated, they will say things like "I don't ever want to do that again" or "I can't afford to do that again." Sometimes they just can't afford it, but sometimes there is a resentment in their tone of voice that they did something against their will or against their better judgement. To me, this is a failed case. The implants may be just fine, but the quality of life that the implants were supposed to provide is not there because the patient feels cheated.

I try very hard to avoid situations like this because it also makes me feel bad. I try to listen very closely to everything a patient says to me to uncover any hidden resistances. However, it is ultimately up to you as the patient to make an informed decision. I think it is important in this process to also listen to your own inner voice. Sometimes in life, there are priorities that override what someone outside your life might consider a high priority. These are things only you can say.

Conversely, it is also possible for someone to avoid dental implants due to some underlying fears about surgery or about the possibilities of implant failure. In spite of what I said earlier, I don't think fear is a good reason to avoid treatment. I know this sounds confusing; it can be a fine line between the resentment felt if you feel you are being "pushed" into something you just don't want and needing a little nudge to overcome a fear you have of getting something that you really do want.

I bring these things up because I think that disappointment with a treatment often is the result of an incomplete decision process. I think that if you consider the emotional side of your treatment, you will come to know what you really want. Whatever you decide, just be sure that it is your decision and not what someone else wants. If you know this going in, you will be ready to fully appreciate what your dental implants can contribute to your quality of life.

Find more information on implants and other dental subjects on my website, Toothhaven.com. You can also follow me on Facebook (https://www.facebook.com/toothhaven) and Twitter (https://twitter.com/sjbrazis).

I hope this book has been useful to you. If you have enjoyed learning about dental implants, please log onto Amazon.com and leave a review of my book to help others find and enjoy this information.

Glossary

A

Abutment—this is used in the context of a fixed bridge (the "abutment teeth" referring to the teeth supporting the bridge), partial removable dentures (the "abutment teeth" referring to the teeth supporting the partial), and in implants (used to attach a crown, bridge, or removable denture to the dental implant fixture)

Abutment screw—the screw used to secure the abutment to the implant body

Adjunctive procedures—procedures used in conjunction with another to increase the chance of success of the main procedure

Allograft—a tissue graft from a donor of the same species as the recipient (but not genetically identical)

Alloplastic graft—grafts using non-biologic material such as metal, ceramic, and plastic. Bone grafting uses a flexible hydrogel-hydroxyapatite (HA) composite that has a mineral to organic matrix ratio, approximating that of human bone

Analog Implant—a manufactured device that is embedded in the operative model and is used during fabrication of the laboratory prosthetics to duplicate the shape and position of the implant body

Autograft—autologous or autogenous bone grafting involves utilizing bone obtained from same individual receiving the graft

B

Bite impression—an impression of upper and lower teeth together where the patient bites into a tray with impression material on both sides to register the position of upper and lower teeth in a closed bite

Bone augmentation—increase in bone dimensions by addition of material or tissue

Bridge—dental bridges literally bridge the gap created by one or more missing teeth. A bridge is made up of two or more crowns for the teeth on either side of the gap (these two or more anchoring teeth are called abutment teeth) and a false tooth/teeth in between called a pontic

Bruxism—the involuntary or habitual grinding of the teeth, typically during sleep

C

Caries, Carious lesion, Cavity—cavity formation in teeth caused by bacteria that attach to teeth and form acids in the presence of sucrose, other sugars, and refined starches; tooth decay

CAT scan—computed tomography, more commonly known as a CT or CAT scan, is a diagnostic medical test that, like traditional x-rays, produces multiple images or pictures of the inside of the body. The cross-sectional images generated during a CT scan can be reformatted in multiple planes, and can even generate three-dimensional images

CBCT scan—Cone beam computed tomography (or CBCT, also referred to as C-arm CT, cone beam volume CT, or flat panel CT) is a medical imaging technique consisting of x-ray computed tomography where the x-rays are divergent, forming a cone. CBCT has become increasingly important in treatment planning and diagnosis in implant dentistry and interventional radiology (IR), among other things. Perhaps because of the increased access to such technology, CBCT scanners are now finding many uses in dentistry, such as in the fields of oral surgery, endodontics and orthodontics

Congenital—of or relating to a condition present at birth, whether inherited or caused by the environment, especially the uterine environment

Contraindication—a specific situation in which a drug, procedure, or surgery should not be used because it may be harmful to the person

There are two types of contraindications:

Relative contraindication means that caution should be used when two drugs or procedures are used together (it is acceptable to do so if the benefits outweigh the risk).

Absolute contraindication means that event or substance could cause a life-threatening situation. A procedure or medicine that falls under this category should be avoided.

Composite resin—dental composite resins are types of synthetic resins which are used in dentistry as restorative material or adhesives (cements). Synthetic resins evolved as restorative materials since they were insoluble, aesthetic, insensitive to dehydration, easy to manipulate and reasonably inexpensive. Composite resins are most commonly composed of Bis-GMA and other dimethacrylate monomers (TEGMA, UDMA, HDDMA), a filler material such as silica, and in most current applications, a photo initiator

Crown—a dental crown is a tooth-shaped "cap" that is placed over a tooth to restore its shape and size, strength, and improve its appearance. The crowns, when cemented into place, fully encase the entire visible portion of a tooth that lies at and above the gum line

Custom abutment—an implant abutment that is constructed specifically for a particular case in order to place the final crown at an angle to the implant body

D

Dental Bonding—is a dental procedure in which a dentist applies a tooth-colored resin material (a durable plastic material) and cures it with visible, blue light. This ultimately "bonds" the material to the tooth or to the metal of a crown, post or implant abutment

Dental implant—a replacement for the root or roots of a tooth. Like tooth roots, dental implants are secured in the jawbone and are not visible once surgically placed. They are used to secure crowns (the parts of teeth seen in the mouth), bridgework, or dentures by a variety of means. They are made of titanium, which is lightweight, strong and biocompatible, which means that it is not rejected by the body

Dental impression—a negative imprint of hard (teeth) and soft tissues in the mouth from which a positive reproduction (or cast) can be formed

Dental prosthesis—an intraoral (inside the mouth) prosthesis used to restore (reconstruct) intraoral defects such as missing teeth, missing parts of teeth, and missing soft or hard structures of the jaw and palate

Denture—a removable plate (full denture) or frame (partial denture) holding one or more artificial teeth

E

Extraction socket—the space left in the bone by the extraction of a tooth

F

Foramen—an opening, hole, or passage, especially in a bone

H

Healing cap—a capped screw used to seal off the interior of an implant body, which can be unscrewed to allow access to the implant body for restoration later

Hydoxyapatite—a mineral of the apatite group that is the main inorganic constituent of tooth enamel and bone

I

Impression coping—a part supplied by implant manufacturers to allow the dentist to replicate the position of an implant body in the dental model used by the laboratory to produce the finished restoration, and which can then be transferred to the patient

M

Mandibular—of or pertaining to the lower jaw

Mandibular canal—a canal in the mandible (lower jaw) containing the nerves and blood vessels that supply the jaw bone and lower teeth

Maxillary—of or pertaining to the upper jaw

O

Occlusal guard—a plastic device made by the dental laboratory from an impression made by the dentist that fits over the biting surfaces of either the upper or lower arch to prevent the patient from grinding or clenching their teeth

Osseointegration—refers to a direct structural and functional connection between ordered, living bone and the surface of a load-carrying implant. Currently, an implant is considered as osseointegrated when there is no progressive relative movement between the implant and the bone with which it has direct contact

Osteonecrosis—a disease resulting from the temporary or permanent loss of blood supply to the bones. Without blood, the bone tissue dies. Osteonecrosis is also known as avascular necrosis, aseptic necrosis, and ischemic necrosis

Osteoporosis—the body constantly absorbs and replaces bone tissue; with osteoporosis, new bone creation doesn't keep up with old bone removal. Osteoporosis causes bones to become weak and brittle—so brittle that a fall or even mild stresses like bending over or coughing can cause a fracture

OTC—referring to medications means over the counter (no prescription needed)

P

Periodontal—literally means "around teeth." Periodontal diseases are infections of the structures around the teeth, which include the gums, periodontal ligament and alveolar bone

Plaque—dental plaque is a biofilm or mass of bacteria that grows on surfaces within the mouth. It is a sticky, colorless deposit at first, but when it forms tartar, it is brown or pale yellow and commonly found between the teeth, front of teeth, behind teeth, on chewing surface, along the gumline, or below the gumline cervical margins

Pontic—an artificial (false) tooth, usually attached to a dental prosthesis, that replaces a missing tooth

S

Sinus cavity—paranasal sinuses are a group of four paired air-filled spaces that surround the nasal cavity. The maxillary sinuses are located under the eyes, the frontal sinuses are above the eyes, the ethmoidal sinuses are between the eyes, and the sphenoidal sinuses are behind the eyes

Sinus lift—surgery that adds bone to the upper jaw in the area of the molars and premolars. It's sometimes called a sinus augmentation. The bone is added between the jaw and the maxillary sinuses, which are on either side of the nose

Space maintainer—helps "hold space" for permanent teeth

Stayplate—also called temporary partial dentures or "flippers." A stayplate will replace the missing tooth or teeth and can assist you with your chewing and/or speaking until your permanent prosthesis (dental implant, fixed bridge, or removable denture) is delivered

Stone model—a dental model is used in dentistry so the dentist can have an exact replica of the patient's teeth, gingiva, and surrounding tissues in the mouth. It can be used for studying purposes to determine the patient's course of treatment. It can also be used for the fabrication of dental prostheses like implant restorations, fixed bridges, crowns, and dentures

Systemic—affecting the entire body, rather than a single organ or body part

T

Titanium—commercially pure titanium has acceptable mechanical properties (especially its ability to osseointegrate) and has been used for orthopedic and dental implants

TMD—temporomandibular disorder, referring to problems inside the temporomandibular joint and the muscles attached to it

TMJ—temporomandibular joint, the only bilateral joint in the body. The mandible bone is connected to a joint on both sides of the body simultaneously, and these bilateral joints must work in harmony

V

Vertical dimension—Vertical dimension of occlusion, or VDO, also known as occlusal vertical dimension (OVD), is a term used in dentistry to indicate the superior-inferior (upper-lower) relationship of the maxilla and the mandible when the teeth are situated in maximum intercuspation (teeth are biting together)

About the Author

Dr. Steven J. Brazis attended dental school at the University of the Pacific School of Dentistry in San Francisco and graduated in 1973. He bought his current practice in 1995 and has had a very successful and fulfilling career here with an excellent and very loyal staff.

Dr. Brazis is a member of the American Dental Association, the California Dental Association, and the Sacramento District Dental Society. He is a past member of the San Francisco Dental Society, where he also served a term on the Curriculum Committee, responsible for the continuing education programs for the society.

Dr. Brazis practices all phases of general dentistry and has had extensive experience in the advancing technological aspects of dentistry. What he enjoys most is the sense of fulfillment of helping someone achieve their best smile, employing the latest technology available to the dental field.

He has five grown children and three grandsons. His interests are mostly outdoor sports and photography. He loves backpacking and getting up into the high country of the Sierra Nevada Mountains. He has climbed almost all of the peaks in the Sierra Nevada range between Mt. Whitney and Yosemite at various times over the past 40 years.

His contact information is:

5030 J Street, Ste. 302
Sacramento, CA 95819
(916) 731-5151
sjbrazis@toothhaven.com